Rebuild & Thrive

Vol. 1

CHAIR WORKOUTS

TO IMPROVE POSTURE, ENHANCE INDEPENDENCE, AND LOSE WEIGHT

for Seniors Over 70

DR. HAMRICK NELSON

Disclaimer

The exercises and information presented in this book are designed to promote health, mobility, and well-being, particularly for seniors. However, it's important to remember that everyone's body is different, and what works well for one person may not be suitable for another. Before starting any new exercise program, especially if you have any pre-existing medical conditions or concerns, please consult with your doctor or healthcare provider to ensure these routines are safe for you.

While every effort has been made to ensure that the exercises are easy to follow and safe, your health and safety are our top priority. It's important to listen to your body—if you experience any discomfort or pain while performing any exercise, stop immediately and seek guidance from a healthcare professional. This book is intended to be a helpful guide, but it should not replace professional medical advice.

Dr. Hamrick Nelson and the team are committed to your well-being and encourage you to approach these exercises with care, patience, and an understanding of your body's needs.

The goal is to help you live a healthier, more active life, one step—or chair exercise—at a time.

Table of Contents

ABOUT THE AUTHOR

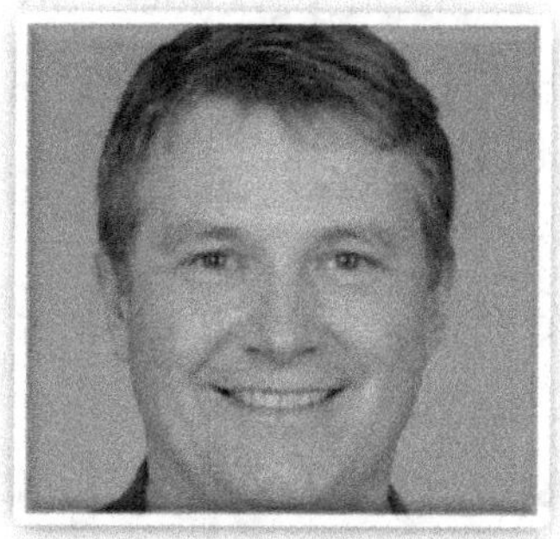 Dr. Hamrick Nelson is a leading voice in fitness and wellness, with a deep passion for helping individuals of all ages live healthier, more active lives. With over two decades of experience in the health and fitness industry, Dr. Nelson has dedicated his career to promoting accessible exercise routines for people at every stage of life. His approach is rooted in the belief that movement is for everyone, regardless of age or physical limitations.

While Dr. Nelson's work spans a wide range of fitness disciplines, he has a special focus on supporting seniors—particularly those over 70. Through his extensive research and hands-on experience, he understands the unique challenges faced by older adults, and he's made it his mission to help them maintain their independence, strength, and vitality. He combines practical knowledge with compassion, creating tailored fitness programs that prioritize safety and long-term health benefits.

Holding advanced degrees in physical therapy and exercise science, Dr. Nelson has worked with countless individuals to enhance their mobility, flexibility, and overall well-being. His books, workshops, and speaking engagements reflect his commitment to helping people of all ages—whether young or senior—stay fit, feel strong, and live life to the fullest.

In *Rebuild & Thrive Vol. 1,* Dr. Nelson focuses on providing seniors, especially those over 70, with simple, effective chair exercises that are designed to improve strength, flexibility, and balance. His program offers an approachable, supportive path to better health, empowering older adults to continue thriving well into their golden years.

What Others Are Saying...

Janet R., 71 years' old

After reading about Mary's experience in this book, I finally felt confident enough to start chair exercises. Like Mary, I've struggled with mobility after surgery, and I thought my best days were behind me. But after following the program, I'm moving more freely and feeling stronger than I have in years. The exercises are simple but so effective.

John S., 74 years' old

This book has been a game changer for me. The exercises are clearly explained, and the step-by-step approach makes it easy to get started. I've lost a few pounds and feel stronger overall. Plus, I love that the exercises can be done from the comfort of a chair—no gym required.

George M., 76 years' old

Bill's story resonated with me. I used to be active, but age has slowed me down, and I've been worried about my health. Seeing how Bill regained his strength and confidence motivated me to try the exercises in this book. I've already noticed improvements in my posture and balance, and I feel more confident with each passing week.

Sarah K., 68 years' old

Mary's journey was the push I needed to get started. I've been dealing with chronic knee pain, and I was hesitant to start any form of exercise. However, after reading how Mary regained her independence, I gave the chair exercises a try. Now, not only is my pain more manageable, but I've also lost a few pounds and feel more energetic. This book has been a lifesaver.

Linda P., 69 years' old

I never thought simple chair exercises could make such a big difference! This book is so easy to follow, and the exercises are perfect for someone like me who's looking for gentle but effective ways to stay fit. I've noticed better flexibility and less joint pain after just a few weeks. I highly recommend this book to anyone looking for a low-impact way to stay active.

INTRODUCTION

Staying active as we age is more than just maintaining physical health; it is also essential for keeping independence, improving mobility, and assuring a higher quality of life. While aging is a normal process, the loss of physical strength, flexibility, and balance does not have to be permanent. Regardless of age, deliberate, low-impact movement can help us reclaim control of our health and well-being. ***"Rebuild & Thrive Vol. 1"*** is intended to provide seniors and people of all ages with the tools they need to stay healthy, active, and independent.

As you read through these pages, you'll see that the path to a healthier, more agile body doesn't involve expensive equipment or rigorous training regimes. All that is required is a chair, some willingness, and careful implementation of the ideas and exercises detailed in this book. Whether you want to lose weight, gain strength, or improve your posture, flexibility, or balance, chair workouts are a safe, effective, and simple choice that you can incorporate into your daily routine.

Chair exercises are extremely versatile, making them appropriate for a wide range of fitness levels and physical ailments. While this book is specifically designed for seniors over the age of 70, chair-based workouts can benefit anybody, from those just starting in fitness to seasoned exercisers wishing to improve their current regimen.

Chair exercises have a unique ability to reduce joint strain, making them a great choice for people suffering from arthritis, joint discomfort, or limited mobility. Furthermore, they provide much-needed stability to seniors who are at a higher danger of falling. These exercises, which incorporate movements that enhance core strength, balance, and flexibility, can help reduce the chance of injury while also increasing general physical health.

For people who have struggled with their weight or felt limited by age or disease, these exercises provide a gentle, long-term strategy to shed weight and enhance heart health. While they may appear easy, these workouts are particularly designed to activate important muscle groups, increase metabolism, and promote circulation.

Meet Mary, a 72-year-old retired schoolteacher who has always maintained an active lifestyle. However, following a knee injury and subsequent surgery, she found herself with limited mobility. Frustrated by her limits, she began to worry about losing her independence. That's when Mary came upon chair workouts. She was at first doubtful about the effectiveness of a sitting workout, but she was quickly surprised by the results. Following the method provided in this book, Mary gradually regained her strength and confidence. Within a few months, she was not only able to move more easily, but she had also lost 15 pounds.

"Chair exercises gave me back something I thought I'd lost forever—my independence," Mary said. "I can move more easily today, and I feel stronger every day. I've even started walking longer distances again!"

Mary's story isn't unique. Many seniors, including her, have discovered that including chair exercises in their daily routine can result in significant benefits in both physical health and emotional well-being. The simple yet powerful exercises in this book are designed to help people like Mary rehabilitate from injury while simultaneously regaining control of their lives, one movement at a time.

That's not all; learn from what Bill has to say after going through a difficult period as an aged person. *Bill, a 74-year-old veteran, was originally apprehensive about attempting chair exercises. He had been an athlete his entire life and struggled with the prospect of having to rely on a chair for support during his training. However, after a heart attack, his doctor strongly advised him to incorporate low-impact activities into his daily routine.*

With his family's encouragement, Bill began performing the strength-building exercises recommended in this book. Within a few weeks, his posture improved significantly, as did his endurance.

His enhanced strength has increased his confidence in his movements, lowering his danger of falling and giving him more energy to pursue his hobbies.

This book provides step-by-step guidance to a range of workouts and routines that are simple to follow, extremely effective, and, most importantly, safe for anyone over 70. Each chapter has been carefully developed to meet the special needs of seniors while also allowing for changes, so people of all ages and fitness levels can benefit.

In the first several chapters, we'll go over the essential principles of chair exercises. You'll learn about the benefits of sitting workouts and why they're a great place to start for people who have mobility issues, balance issues, or limited fitness experience. This book also includes important safety guidelines to help you avoid injuries throughout your workouts.

Warming up is essential, especially as we age, and in this book, you'll learn easy, effective warm-up activities that get your muscles ready for movement. You'll then graduate to specialized weight reduction activities that assist burn calories and enhance cardiovascular health while seated, with much more to learn as you progress through your studies.

As you read through the exercises and routines in this book, keep in mind the importance of consistency. Chair exercises are most effective when done regularly; over time, you will see gains in your strength, flexibility, balance, and overall health. The workouts are designed in such a way that you can grow at your own pace. I advise you to listen to your body and alter the workouts as necessary.

Each chapter builds on the last, therefore it's best to read the book in order. However, feel free to repeat previous exercises or combine programs to suit your own needs.

This book is more than simply about physical fitness; it is about regaining control of your life, enhancing your well-being, and feeling empowered to face the future with confidence. The journey to greater health begins here, and I'm delighted to accompany you every step of the way.

CHAPTER 1: KNOWING THE BASIC PRINCIPLES OF CHAIR EXERCISES

For those with limited mobility, especially the elderly, chair exercises provide a low-impact, accessible form of physical activity that may be done while seated in a chair. Strength, flexibility, balance, and cardiovascular health are just a few of the fitness objectives that can be addressed by these workouts, which don't need participants to stand or bear their full body weight. Particularly for people recovering from accidents, managing chronic diseases, or seeking gentle methods to stay active, these chair-supported workouts offer a safe and efficient way to maintain or improve physical fitness.

Chair workouts usually involve seated motions such as torso twists, leg extensions, and arm lifts. They might use the back of a chair, resistance bands, or small weights to give them support when performing standing activities. Chair exercises, despite their simplicity, can be customized to match a variety of fitness levels, from novice to expert, and may offer a full-body workout. Chair exercises are a flexible fitness option for strength growth, flexibility enhancement, and weight loss since they can be customized to meet individual goals.

Although chair exercises have several health benefits, they are best suited for the elderly or people with physical limitations due to their advantages over other forms of exercise. The following explains why chair exercises are unique and offer clear advantages:

1. Fit for all levels of fitness

The fact that chair workouts are suitable for individuals of all fitness levels—especially those who have trouble standing or engaging in high-impact activities—is one of their most noteworthy advantages. For people with joint issues, chronic conditions like arthritis, or limited mobility, traditional forms of exercise like jogging, leaping, or lifting weights might be challenging. Conversely, chair workouts offer a comfortable setting where movements are performed while seated, significantly reducing the tension on muscles, joints, and bones.

Chair exercises offer an introduction to physical activity without the risk of injury or overexertion for beginners or those getting back into shape after a long break. They enable people to gradually improve their fitness and build confidence without having to perform increasingly challenging or taxing exercises.

2. Safety and reduced injury risk

Chair workouts offer a major benefit in terms of safety, which is a top priority for many elderly people and people with health issues. Sitting exercises lower the risk of falling or losing balance, which is particularly advantageous for people with weak muscles or poor coordination. This is crucial since falls are a major cause of injuries among the elderly, often leading to fractures or other serious issues.

These exercises are also gentler on the body because of the chair's supportive structure, which lessens the strain on bones and joints. People with osteoporosis or arthritis can remain active with chair workouts without experiencing any pain or discomfort. Chair exercises are safe for persons with medical conditions or past injuries because of the controlled movements, which also reduce the risk of overextending muscles or tendons.

3. Flexibility in meeting personal demands

The adaptability of chair exercises is among its most fascinating features. These exercises can easily be modified to accommodate different people's needs. The level of difficulty and intensity of chair exercises can be changed to accommodate total beginners, surgical patients, or anyone seeking a more difficult workout.

Certain movements can be made more difficult, for instance, by using resistance bands or small hand weights; those who require more help can stick to easy, moderate activities. With this method, chair exercises can target a variety of fitness goals, such as increasing flexibility and strength, all within the same framework.

Additionally, chair workouts can be tailored to focus on certain body parts, such as the arms, legs, or core. They are therefore particularly useful for those who wish to focus on a particular area without putting undue effort on other body parts. For instance, a person recuperating from knee surgery can concentrate on strengthening their upper body without standing or exerting weight on their lower body.

4. Easy access and minimal equipment needs

Chair exercises also have the benefit of being convenient. As long as there is a sturdy chair available, they can be performed almost anywhere. They are a desirable alternative for those who might find it difficult to access conventional training facilities because they don't require a gym membership or specialized equipment.

For seniors who like to work out at home, chair exercises are ideal. A strong chair is all you need; you can add other equipment, such as resistance bands or light weights, for variation, but they are not necessary. Because of this, chair workouts are simple and affordable to incorporate into a routine, regardless of the person's living situation.

People who live in apartments assisted living facilities, or smaller homes can benefit from chair exercises because they are portable and can be done in small spaces. Seniors and those with limited mobility can stay active without the logistical problems that come with larger training sets because of the minimal space and equipment requirements.

5. Assimilation into everyday life

One clear benefit of chair workouts is that they are simple to include in daily routines. Chair exercises can often be done in short bursts throughout the day, unlike more complex fitness routines that may require dedicated time and attention. Elderly persons and those with hectic schedules may find it easier to maintain a regular physical activity routine if they can divide their workouts into smaller chunks.

For instance, one could stretch their upper body while seated at a desk or dining table, or perform a series of leg lifts while watching television. Because there is no need to schedule a substantial amount of time for exercise, this flexibility makes it simpler to stick to a routine. Chair workouts are a long-term fitness option since they can be integrated into everyday activities.

6. Effective but low-impact

Chair exercises can be very beneficial for increasing strength, flexibility, and cardiovascular fitness even though they are low-impact and gentle on the joints. Chair exercises can provide a challenging and comprehensive workout with the right movements and adjustments, despite the common misconception that they cannot be as strenuous as standing exercises.

While seated marches or toe taps can raise the heart rate for an aerobic workout, upper body exercises like sitting bicep curls or seated chest pushes can effectively develop muscle strength. People can still gain muscle and increase their fitness without standing or performing high-intensity movements thanks to chair exercises, which are controlled and enable targeted muscle engagement.

7. Fit for chronic diseases and rehabilitation

The fact that chair exercises can be used by those undergoing rehabilitation or managing long-term medical issues is another important advantage. Conventional exercise regimens often overstress healing muscles, bones, or joints, which can impede recovery or exacerbate symptoms of some diseases. Conversely, chair exercises are gentle enough to be incorporated into a rehabilitation program for individuals recuperating from illnesses, injuries, or surgeries.

Because chair exercises are low-impact and encourage mobility, which is essential for general health, they are beneficial for people with chronic conditions like arthritis, osteoporosis, or cardiovascular disease. Frequent exercise can prevent muscular weakening, increase blood flow, and reduce stiffness—all of which are critical for the management of chronic illnesses. Chair exercises, in particular, offer a safe and efficient way to keep the body moving, preventing the loss of mobility that can happen after extended periods of inactivity.

Because chair exercises help patients build strength, flexibility, and range of motion without placing undue strain on sensitive areas, physical therapists commonly incorporate them into rehabilitation plans. For instance, a person recuperating from hip or knee surgery can gradually increase their level of fitness and get their body ready to resume more conventional forms of exercise by working on strengthening their core or upper body while seated.

8. Encourages self-sufficiency and aging in situ

Maintaining their independence is a top priority for many seniors, and chair exercises can help them remain independent for longer. As people age, their muscle strength, flexibility, and balance may diminish, making everyday tasks like getting out of bed, getting out of a chair, or short walks more challenging. The physical strength needed to perform these tasks on their own is developed and maintained by seniors with the help of chair exercises.

The ability to perform everyday tasks safely and independently is known as functional fitness, and it can be enhanced in older adults by regular chair exercises. This can reduce their fear of falling or getting hurt by boosting their self-confidence. Chair exercises therefore help seniors age in place by enabling them to remain in their homes and communities for extended periods of time without needing a lot of aid.

Additionally, the increased strength and mobility that chair exercises provide can improve seniors' quality of life by enabling them to travel, engage in hobbies, and enjoy social activities. Elderly people benefit emotionally and physically from this sense of independence, which preserves their autonomy and dignity.

9. Advantages for mental and cognitive health

Chair exercises have clear physical benefits, but it's important to consider their effects on mental health as well. Frequent exercise, even simple chair exercises, has been shown to reduce stress, anxiety, and depression symptoms. Endorphins, which are natural mood enhancers that enhance feelings of well-being, are released when you exercise. Seniors who are more likely to experience feelings of loneliness or isolation may benefit from chair exercises.

Chair workouts have cognitive advantages in addition to enhancing mental health. Chair workouts require coordination and focus for many of their actions, which can enhance and stimulate cognitive performance. For instance, exercises that include raising the legs and moving the arms force participants to concentrate on coordinating many motions simultaneously, which enhances mental clarity.

Because frequent mental engagement helps prevent cognitive decline and increase memory, this cognitive stimulation is especially important for the elderly. Chair exercises can serve as a kind of moving meditation, promoting relaxation and stress reduction when paired with deliberate movement and focused breathing. Including chair exercises in a senior's routine can help them relax both physically and mentally, improving their overall quality of life if they have trouble sleeping or are under a lot of stress.

10. Encourages engagement in groups and social interaction

Chair exercises are typically performed in groups, such as in community centers, senior living facilities, or online fitness programs, although they can also be done alone. An extra advantage of chair workouts is that they encourage social interaction and connection. Many elderly people think that maintaining social connections is essential to their mental and emotional well-being. Exercise groups foster a sense of support and camaraderie that keeps people motivated and responsible for their fitness routines.

In addition to improving the experience and reducing feelings of loneliness, exercising with others can also foster a vibrant and pleasurable atmosphere. Seniors who live alone or far from family have the chance to meet new people, make friends, and exchange experiences through chair exercise classes. By lowering emotions of loneliness, this social interaction can promote better mental health.

Online groups or virtual chair workouts might make you feel more connected and motivated, even if you prefer to work out at home. By joining a virtual club, people can work out from the comfort of their homes and stay encouraged and engaged. Chair workouts can be more enjoyable and sustainable as part of a healthy lifestyle since these cultures value friendship and common objectives.

11. Simple to adapt and customize

The ability to easily adapt and customize chair workouts to each person's needs and objectives is another important benefit. Chair exercises offer a flexible framework that may be customized to a person's fitness level, physical limitations, and personal preferences, regardless of how long they have been exercising.

For instance, people with joint discomfort or mobility issues could stick to low-impact, gentler exercises that focus on flexibility and mobility, while more experienced participants can up the ante with weights, resistance bands, or more dynamic routines. Because of their adaptability, chair exercises can keep people challenged and help them get fitter as their fitness levels rise.

Chair exercises can be made to focus on particular health problems, such as strengthening core muscles, reducing back pain, or improving posture. Chair workouts are a very flexible option for anyone attempting to reach particular fitness objectives without putting undue strain on their body because of their adaptability. Because chair workouts let users customize the exercises to suit their own needs, they promote a sense of independence and self-empowerment in fitness.

Chair workouts are an excellent option for people of all fitness levels, especially seniors and those with mobility challenges because they offer several specialized benefits. Numerous factors, such as accessibility, safety, versatility, and convenience, make chair exercises advantageous. By offering a low-impact, efficient method of increasing strength, flexibility, and overall fitness, chair exercises help people maintain their independence, enhance their physical and mental well-being, and lead healthier lives. Chair exercises offer a useful, sustainable, and pleasurable approach to staying active and healthy, whether they are performed in groups or alone, at home, or in the community.

Benefits To Mental And Physical Health

For seniors, especially those with restricted mobility or balance issues, chair workouts offer a novel and efficient way to get moving. Engaging in these activities can significantly enhance one's mental and physical health and promote a healthier way of living. *We'll examine the main advantages of chair workouts for seniors' physical and mental health below:*

Benefits to Physical Health:

1. **Improved stamina and strength:** Increased muscular strength and endurance are one of the main advantages of chair exercises. Seniors can benefit from regular chair exercises that increase muscle tone, especially in the upper and lower body. Seniors can preserve functional strength by performing exercises that focus on important muscular areas, such as leg lifts, chest presses, and sitting bicep curls. This is necessary for daily activities including getting out of a chair, going upstairs, and carrying groceries.

2. **Greater adaptability:** Age-related losses in flexibility lead to stiffness and an increased risk of injury. Stretching motions used in chair exercises can increase flexibility in key areas such as the shoulders, hips, and back. Seniors can do everyday tasks more comfortably by maintaining their

range of motion with the help of poses like the seated forward bend and seated twists.

3. **Improved coordination and balance:** Elderly people are particularly concerned about falls because many of them cause significant injuries. Chair exercises that test stability can improve coordination and balance. Balance requires core stability, which is enhanced by exercises like side reaches and sitting leg raises. Seniors who perform these movements daily can increase their overall stability and reduce their chance of falling.

4. **Controlling weight:** Weight management requires regular activity, particularly while seated. For seniors who wish to lose weight or maintain a healthy weight, chair exercises can increase calorie expenditure. Exercises that are more dynamic, such as leg extensions or sitting marching, can raise heart rates and help people lose weight. Additionally, maintaining a healthy weight reduces your chance of contracting long-term illnesses like diabetes and heart disease.

5. **Heart health:** By increasing heart rate and circulation, chair exercises improve cardiovascular fitness. Easy exercises like arm circles and seated marches can increase heart rate and strengthen the heart. Engaging in these activities regularly

can help reduce the risk of heart disease, improve cholesterol levels, and lower blood pressure.

6. **Pain management and joint health:** Joint stiffness and discomfort are typical in older adults and are frequently brought on by conditions like arthritis. Chair workouts can provide gentle motions that improve joint health and lubricate the joints. Seniors' quality of life can be enhanced by using low-impact exercises and seated stretching to alleviate pain and stiffness. Maintaining joint function requires regular mobility, which can also help to lessen the severity of arthritis symptoms.

Advantages of Mental Health

1. **Decreased signs of anxiety and despair:** It has been demonstrated that physical activity, including chair exercises, enhances mental wellness. Frequent exercise helps reduce emotions of worry and hopelessness by releasing endorphins, the body's natural mood enhancers. Elderly people may find that chair exercises help them feel happier and less depressed or lonely.

2. **Improved mental abilities:** A growing body of research suggests that physical activity can enhance elderly adults' cognitive abilities. Frequent exercise increases blood flow to

the brain, which enhances neuroplasticity and encourages the growth of new brain cells. Because chair exercises work both the body and the mind, they can be a useful tool for seniors, especially when memory or coordination issues are added to physical activity.

3. **Increased confidence and self-worth:** Completing chair exercises can boost confidence and self-esteem while also giving one a sense of accomplishment. Seniors may feel more capable of performing daily tasks when their strength, flexibility, and balance improve via exercise. People may be inspired to attempt new things, socialize more, and take part in community events as a result of their improved confidence.

4. **Social engagement and communication:** Group chair exercise sessions are a source of inspiration and enjoyment for many senior individuals. People can engage with one another in these social settings, fostering a feeling of community and belonging. Engaging in physical activity with people can improve mental health by reducing feelings of loneliness and isolation. Elders can talk about their experiences, support one another, and celebrate their accomplishments in a supportive setting during group sessions.

5. **Relaxation and stress reduction:** Chair exercises and other regular physical activities are effective ways to reduce stress. Neurotransmitters that help control mood are released more when you exercise, which reduces stress and anxiety. Additionally, breathing exercises that promote relaxation may be incorporated with chair exercises to help seniors manage their stress levels. Elderly people can achieve inner calm and center themselves in the face of everyday problems by practicing mindfulness by concentrating on their breathing and movement.

6. **Enhanced life quality:** Chair exercises improve one's quality of life by offering benefits to one's physical and mental health. Seniors may find it simpler to engage in social activities, pursue hobbies, and fully enjoy life as their strength, flexibility, and confidence increase. Frequent exercise can help seniors stay independent for longer by giving them the confidence they need to lead happier, more active lives.

Chair exercises are a great addition to any fitness program since they offer seniors several physical and mental health advantages. By enhancing their strength, flexibility, balance, and cardiovascular health, these activities help seniors become more independent and feel better overall. The overall advantages of regular physical activity are further highlighted by the mental health advantages, which include decreased depression symptoms, enhanced cognitive performance, and increased social interaction.

Chair exercises are a fun, safe, and efficient way for seniors to stay active and thrive in their golden years if they want to improve their health. Elderly people can enjoy happier, healthier, and more fulfilling lives as more of them become aware of the advantages of chair exercises.

Influence On Controlling Weight

Controlling one's weight is crucial for preserving general health, especially for those over 70. Maintaining a healthy weight becomes increasingly challenging as we age because our metabolism slows down. Weight management can be greatly impacted by regular exercise, particularly chair exercises.

Maintaining a healthy body weight by combining exercise and diet is known as weight management. Because being overweight raises the risk of chronic diseases including diabetes, heart disease, and joint problems, weight control is particularly crucial for seniors. Conversely, being underweight may lead to immune system impairment, malnourishment, and muscle weakness. Therefore, striking the right balance is essential.

How Exercises in Chairs Aid with Weight Management

1. **Caloric expenditure:** Burning more calories than you consume is one of the best ways to lose weight. Chair exercises can nevertheless make a substantial contribution to total caloric expenditure, even though they don't burn as many calories as high-impact activities. Leg lifts, upper body movements, and seated marching all increase heart rate and muscular activation, which burns calories. Seniors can

raise their physical activity levels without going overboard with chair exercises, which are both safe and effective.

2. **Increasing muscle mass:** The aging-related normal loss of muscular mass is known as sarcopenia. A slower metabolism brought on by less muscle mass may make it more challenging to maintain a healthy weight. Strength training-focused chair workouts, like seated chest presses and bicep curls, help build and maintain muscle mass. Gaining muscle improves your overall body composition and helps you reach a healthy weight in addition to increasing your resting calorie expenditure.

3. **Increasing metabolism:** Frequent exercise, particularly chair exercises, can enhance metabolic performance. A more efficient metabolism is the outcome of exercise, which improves metabolic pathways that help break down glucose and fat. For seniors in particular, this is helpful because a higher metabolic rate can help with weight loss or management and reduce the risk of health issues associated with weight.

4. **Raising levels of physical activity:** Chair exercises could be a starting point for increased physical activity. Beginning with chair exercises might help seniors who may have been sedentary gain confidence and endurance so they can

participate in more activities outside of their exercise regimen. Elderly people may be encouraged to undertake new physical activities as their strength and mobility increase, which will help them with their weight management efforts.

5. **Sustainability and accessibility:** Convenience is one of the main advantages of chair exercises. Common exercises might be challenging for many seniors who have chronic pain or mobility problems. Because chair workouts may be done at home, maintaining a routine is much simpler. These exercises' simplicity of integration into daily life encourages dedication to a regular exercise regimen, which is essential for managing weight.

People over 70 can efficiently maintain their weight with chair exercises. Seniors can improve their metabolism, muscle mass, calorie expenditure, and overall levels of physical activity by implementing these easy activities into their daily routines. Although maintaining a healthy weight might be challenging, seniors can overcome this important aspect of their health with the right resources, support, and perseverance.

Safety Precautions And Guidance For Seniors

Continuing to be physically active as we age is essential for enhancing our independence, health, and general well-being. But putting safety first is essential to avoiding accidents and guaranteeing a wonderful day. *Here are comprehensive safety guidelines and recommendations for senior citizens doing chair exercises:*

1. Seniors should speak with their healthcare professional before starting a new exercise program. An individual's health, medications, and physical capabilities can be assessed by a physician or physical therapist, who can then offer customized advice on suitable exercises and any necessary adjustments. For elderly people with long-term conditions like arthritis, heart disease, or balance issues, this stage is crucial.

2. Exercise chairs must be sturdy, well-made, and ideally wheel-free. When a senior sit in a chair, their feet should be flat on the floor. This encourages proper balance and posture. When working out, a chair with a high back provides stability and support. It improves comfort and lessens back strain. People with weaker muscles may find it easier to sit and stand up in chairs with armrests.

3. Establishing a secure training environment is essential to preventing accidents and falls. To lessen tripping dangers, clear the area surrounding the chair of any clutter, loose carpets, or obstructions. To improve safety and visibility, make sure the exercise area is well-lit. To light the entire space, think about using overhead lights or bright, natural lighting. Try to work out on non-slip surfaces wherever possible. Make sure the carpet is firmly fastened to the floor if you plan to use one.

4. The comfort and safety of chair workouts can be significantly impacted by wearing the proper clothing and footwear. Put on loose-fitting clothing that doesn't restrict your movement. Steer clear of anything that hinders movement, such as long gowns that could get entangled or tight jeans. Put on traction-enhancing, supportive, non-slip shoes. Wearing flip-flops or slippers can make it more likely that you will slip.

5. For seniors in particular, warming up and cooling down are crucial components of any workout regimen. The body is prepared for an exercise with a 5–10 minute warm-up. Blood flow to muscles and joints can be improved with mild exercises like wrist circles, shoulder rolls, and seated marches. After completing the chair exercises, take a few

minutes to stretch and let your pulse rate drop. This improves flexibility and prevents muscle soreness.

6. Elderly people should be conscious of their bodies and know how important it is to pay attention to their feelings when exercising. You must stop working out right away if it causes you any pain or discomfort. Usually, pain is a sign that something is amiss and that continuing could be harmful. Not everyone will benefit from every workout. It is OK for seniors to modify routines to fit their comfort level. For instance, a sitting leg slide can be a better option if a leg lift is too challenging.

7. Everyone needs to drink enough water, but seniors need to pay particular attention because they might not experience thirst even though their bodies need fluids. Seniors should be encouraged to drink a glass of water before starting an exercise regimen and to rehydrate afterward. Drink plenty of water if your workout lasts more than an hour.

8. Proper breathing during exercise can enhance both safety and performance. When exercising, seniors should take deep, steady breaths. During simple exercises, breathe in via your nose, and during more challenging ones, expel through your mouth. This technique encourages relaxation and aids in supplying oxygen to the muscles.

9. To improve stability and reduce the risk of falling, chair exercises can be combined with balance training. You may strengthen your core and increase stability by incorporating easy balance exercises into your program, like leg lifts or sitting heel-to-toe movements. Seniors who participate in these activities may eventually feel more secure and self-assured when walking or standing.

10. Exercises done with other people can be enjoyable, motivating, and encouraging. Think about going to a chair exercise class at the gym or community center in your area. Working out with others fosters a sense of belonging and may lead to greater accountability. Make it a fun activity that fosters relationships and improves health by inviting family members to participate in the exercises.

11. For seniors, monitoring their success can be a powerful motivator. Elderly people should be encouraged to maintain an activity diary where they can write the kinds of activities they engage in, the time spent on each, and their feelings afterward. People might be encouraged to remain involved by using this record to monitor progress over time.

12. For people who are new to exercising or are unsure about how to proceed safely, getting professional counsel can be

very helpful. Speak with a physical therapist or a qualified trainer with expertise in senior fitness. They can design customized workout plans that guarantee safe and effective actions.

Seniors can reclaim their independence, enhance their quality of life, and maintain good physical condition with chair exercises. But the most important factor should always be safety. Seniors can enjoy a safe and effective fitness program that meets their unique needs and enhances their well-being by heeding these warnings and recommendations. Frequent exercise is crucial for good aging since it enhances mental and social well-being in addition to physical fitness.

Tools And Equipment Needed For Chair Exercises

When using chair exercises to improve your physical fitness, having the right tools and equipment can significantly increase the efficacy of your routine. A few simple items can help make workouts more comfortable, safe, and enjoyable, even though many chair exercises can be performed without any specialized equipment. The essential instruments and equipment that can support seniors' chair exercise routines will be covered in this section.

1. A strong/sturdy chair

A sturdy chair is the most fundamental piece of equipment for chair exercises. This chair ought to be sturdy, comfortable, and height-appropriate. The chair should be made to allow the user to sit with their hips slightly higher than their knees, their feet flat on the floor, and their knees bent at a 90-degree angle. When exercising, this position is crucial for preserving proper balance and posture.

By offering additional support, armrests can facilitate getting in and out of a chair. A straight-backed chair encourages good posture, which is necessary for a variety of exercises.

Non-Slip Surface: To prevent slippage when moving, make sure the chair is on a stable floor or has a non-slip surface.

2. Resistance Bands

Resistance bands are practical and affordable tools that add resistance to chair exercises, boosting stamina and strength. They are suitable for users with different levels of fitness because they are available in a range of resistance levels. Loop bands, flat bands, and tube bands are among the varieties. While tube bands have handles for better grip, loop bands are typically more practical for seated exercises since they can be secured beneath the feet.

Exercises like leg lifts, chest presses, and sitting bicep curls can all be performed using resistance bands. They provide a safe way to increase resistance without running the danger of injury that comes with using heavy weights.

3. Light dumbbells

Another helpful addition to a chair training program is light dumbbells. They can be used in a variety of exercises and are excellent for strengthening the upper body. Pick a weight that is challenging but doable. Depending on their level of strength, seniors may weigh anywhere from one and five pounds.

Select dumbbells that are easy to hold. Some might include rough or rubberized surfaces to keep people from slipping, which is particularly useful for those with weak hands.

Use dumbbells that don't cause pain or strain. It is advised to start with smaller weights and increase them gradually as strength increases.

4. A non-slip surface or yoga mat

Chair exercises can be made safer by using a yoga mat or making sure the surface is non-slip. Slips and falls are avoided by using a mat to cushion the feet. A thicker mat is better suited for sitting activities since it may provide greater padding.

To stop the mat from moving while working out, place it on a level, solid surface.

5. Chair, pillow, or yoga block

During a range of exercises, a firm pillow or yoga block can aid offer comfort and support. To make certain stretches simpler to perform, elevate the legs with a block or pillow. They can also help you maintain proper posture by offering extra support when you're seated. During extended workouts, using a cushion with a firm design may make things more comfortable.

6. A bottle of water

Any workout regimen, including chair exercises, requires proper hydration. Regular hydration breaks are encouraged when water is easily accessible. You can stay hydrated while working out with a small, lightweight water bottle.

7. A towel

During chair workouts, a towel can be used for a variety of purposes. Covering the chair seat with a towel could make sitting more comfortable and supportive. In warmer areas, a towel can also be used to wipe away perspiration and maintain personal hygiene when working out.

8. Audio Equipment or Music

Chair exercises can be made more enjoyable and motivating by using music or an audio device. Energizing music boosts motivation and mood during exercise. Elderly people may find it simpler to finish exercises if they receive guidance and timing from guided audio workouts.

9. Workout Manual or Video Source

The chair exercise experience can be significantly enhanced by having access to an exercise manual or video resource. By ensuring that exercises are performed correctly, visual instruction can help reduce the risk of injury.

Resources with a variety of activities encourage regular participation by keeping routines interesting and captivating. To assist you in setting and achieving your goals, several guides include tracking tools.

10. Supportive Footwear

Proper footwear is crucial for both comfort and safety during chair workouts, even if it isn't technically equipment in the usual sense. Non-slip soles of shoes reduce the risk of falls, particularly while getting up or out of a chair. Well-fitting shoes reduce the chance of discomfort during activity by providing the right amount of support and comfort.

Having the right tools for chair exercises can enhance the experience overall and increase the safety and effectiveness of sessions. In addition to adding variety to exercise regimens, a sturdy chair, resistance bands, light dumbbells, and other helpful equipment also cater to the unique requirements of senior citizens. Seniors can engage more fully in their exercise routines when a safe and comfortable environment is provided, which enhances their physical health, independence, and quality of life. As always, speak with your doctor before starting a new fitness program, particularly if you have any underlying medical conditions.

CHAPTER 2: GETTING STARTED AND WARM-UP EXERCISES

Determine Your Current Fitness Level

Especially for seniors over 70, determining your current level of fitness is a crucial first step in developing a successful exercise program. You can set reasonable goals, adapt your training regimen to your capabilities, and monitor your progress over time by being aware of your current physical condition. Your healthcare provider may be made aware of any particular limitations you may have by this evaluation.

Why should you examine your level of fitness?

1. Everybody has a unique physique, particularly as they get older. By determining your level of fitness, you may adjust your training schedule to meet your unique objectives and limitations.

2. Recognizing your skills and limitations can help you build on them while recognizing your limitations might point you in the direction of areas where you can improve.

3. By assessing your level of fitness, you may create attainable objectives that will motivate you without being too demanding.

4. Frequent evaluations can provide you with motivation and a feeling of accomplishment by allowing you to track your development over time.

5. By identifying possible health hazards or injuries, a thorough evaluation enables you to steer clear of exercises that could exacerbate pre-existing conditions.

When assessing your level of fitness, look at the following key areas:

1. Cardiovascular Endurance: This speaks to the capacity of your heart and lungs to tolerate prolonged physical strain.

How to Evaluate:

The Timed Walk Test is a fundamental method. See how far you can walk in six minutes on a level, straight line (like a track or hallway). A common distance for seniors is between 300 and 400 meters. You can use your treadmill or stationary bike in its place.

2. Muscular Strength: This is the most force that a muscle is capable of producing.

How to Evaluate:

The Chair Stand Test is one method of assessment. Place your arms over your chest and sit on the edge of a stable chair. Get up, then take a 30-second break to sit down. During that time, count the number of times you can stand up. 8 to 12 repeats is typically a good score. Assess your ability to complete sitting bicep curls with small weights for a more difficult test.

3. Flexibility: The range of motion in your muscles and joints is what is known as flexibility.

How to Evaluate:

A great substitute is the Chair Sit and Reach Test. With one foot on the floor and one leg straight out in front of you, sit on the edge of a chair. Reach for your toes on the outstretched leg with both hands. Assess your range of motion beyond your toes. It is considered appropriate for elders to be 2-4 inches past their toes.

4. Balance: Maintaining independence and preventing falls need balance.

How to Evaluate:

A chair can be used to provide support when performing the Single Leg Stand Test. For as long as you can, stand on one leg without touching anything. Aim for at least 10 seconds per leg, ideally.

5. Body Composition: The percentage of fat and non-fat mass in your body is known as your body composition.

How to Evaluate:

Although the most accurate measures require specialized equipment, basic methods like taking your waist circumference can be adequate. An elevated risk of health problems may be indicated by a waist circumference greater than 35 inches for women and 40 inches for men.

Instruments for Evaluation

1. **Fitness Trackers:** Your total level of fitness is influenced by your heart rate, sleep patterns, and daily activity levels, all of which may be usefully determined by wearable fitness trackers.

2. **Mobile Apps:** You can navigate tests and monitor your progress over time with the help of a variety of apps.

3. **Professional Assessment:** Seek advice from a physical therapist or personal trainer who specializes in senior fitness, if at all possible. They can do a comprehensive assessment and create a customized training plan according to your needs.

An essential first step in creating a successful senior exercise program is determining your current level of fitness. Knowing your body composition, physical strength, flexibility, balance, and cardiovascular endurance enables you to set reasonable goals, monitor your progress, and eventually improve your general health and well-being. Keep in mind that everyone has a different path to fitness, so you have to go at your speed.

Establishing Attainable Objectives And Monitoring Results

Setting reasonable objectives and effectively monitoring progress are essential for getting the most out of chair exercises. Any exercise program should include goal-setting since it provides inspiration and guidance. Setting goals aids in maintaining focus on your goals and facilitates the development of a methodical action plan. Setting clear objectives for seniors performing chair exercises can improve their physical well-being, self-esteem, and overall quality of life.

There are two types of goals: short-term and long-term

It just takes a few weeks or months to accomplish short-term objectives. They can keep you motivated and act as stepping stones to more ambitious objectives. More important are long-term objectives, which may take months or even years to accomplish. These goals provide your fitness journey with a broader perspective and let you concentrate on important turning points.

Make sure your goals are realistic, achievable, and suitable for your skill level when setting them, especially for chair exercises. *This is a detailed how-to for creating successful goals:*

1. Before establishing goals, assess your level of fitness. Think about your overall mobility, strength, flexibility, and balance. This assessment will help you set reasonable goals and figure out what is feasible.

2. Think about the aspects of your fitness that you would like to enhance. Do you want to improve your balance, lose weight, or get stronger and more flexible? Setting more targeted goals will be possible if you can identify clear areas of focus.

3. Use the SMART criterion to make sure your goals are effective:

- **Specific:** *State your objectives clearly (e.g., "I want to improve my leg strength").*
- **Measurable:** *Establish benchmarks (e.g., "I will be able to perform 10 seated leg lifts in a row") to monitor your development.*
- **Achievable:** *Make sure your objectives (e.g., "I will increase my seated leg lifts from 5 to 10 within four weeks") are appropriate for your current level of fitness and any limitations.*
- **Relevant:** *Your objectives ought to align with your objectives for general health (e.g., "Improving my strength will help me maintain independence").*

- ***Time-bond:*** *Give yourself a deadline to meet your objectives (e.g., "I will finish this within the next month").*

4. Since life can be unpredictable, it's critical to be flexible. Reevaluate your goals and make any required adjustments if you encounter obstacles or setbacks. Being adaptable keeps you motivated and committed to your training schedule.

Monitoring Your Development

Monitoring your progress is crucial for maintaining motivation and focus once you've set your goals. Tracking your accomplishments enables you to recognize areas that could need more attention while also appreciating your victories. The following are some great methods for monitoring progress:

1. Note your exercises, repetitions, and emotions as you go. By documenting this data, you will be able to track your development over time and learn about your successes.

2. To visually monitor your objectives and advancement, make a progress chart. To monitor particular metrics, such as the number of repetitions or the length of an exercise session, you can utilize charts or graphs. Visual aids that highlight your progress can be incredibly motivating.

3. Break down your long-term objectives into manageable chunks. When you reach each milestone, whether it's improving your performance in a particular activity or sticking to your program, celebrate your successes.

4. Examine your fitness journey regularly. Think about how your objectives have evolved, the challenges you've encountered, and your physical sensations. Reflection can provide you with important insights and let you adjust your objectives as necessary.

5. For accountability and support, tell your loved ones about your objectives and accomplishments. Having a support network might help you stay motivated and follow your workout regimen.

For seniors who engage in chair exercises, a good fitness regimen must include setting reasonable goals and monitoring their progress. You may map out a clear path to achieving your fitness objectives by assessing your present level of fitness, pinpointing particular areas that require improvement, and creating goals based on the SMART criteria.

Including Social Considerations In Chair Exercise Programs

Maintaining excellent health requires physical activity, particularly for elders over 70. Adding social aspects to exercise routines can greatly increase motivation, adherence, and overall well-being as people deal with the problems of aging. Social connections, family involvement, and group sessions foster a sense of accountability, encouragement, and belonging that can significantly influence their fitness path.

The Value of Social Engagement in Exercise

Being socially involved is a fundamental human need. Elderly people, who could feel alone or isolated, should pay particular attention to this. Incorporating family members into fitness regimens or taking part in group exercise classes may help create a positive atmosphere that counteracts negative thinking. Seniors who engage in social activities are more likely to stick with their fitness regimens and benefit from the many physical and mental health advantages that regular exercise offers, according to studies.

1. **Enhanced Motivation:** Working out with other people might increase motivation. In a group setting, participants

can help one another, share challenges, and celebrate successes together. Elderly people may be inspired to overcome suffering or fatigue by this shared experience, knowing that they have a network of support behind them.

2. **Enhanced Accountability:** Family participation or group education can promote accountability. Seniors are less likely to skip a lesson or workout when they are aware that others are counting on them to show up. They may be inspired to maintain consistency by this commitment to others.

3. **Better Mental Health:** Seniors who exercise and socialize might overcome feelings of depression and loneliness. Social interactions, experience sharing, and conversation can all enhance mental health and mood.

Another excellent method to incorporate social aspects into chair exercise routines is through senior-specific group exercise programs. These classes are frequently taught by certified teachers who are aware of the special requirements of senior citizens and can modify exercises to suit varying levels of fitness.

1. **Sessions available:** A range of chair exercise sessions are offered by community centers, gyms, and senior living institutions

2. **Creating a Community:** Attending group activities on a regular basis encourages people to connect with their peers. These exchanges have the potential to grow into friendships over time, providing social support outside of the gym environment. In addition to the physical activity, seniors may look forward to class because of the friendships they form with their peers.

3. **Engaging Teachers:** Trained teachers create a welcoming atmosphere in addition to leading exercises. They can contribute ideas, lead group discussions, and add social elements to the classroom. By encouraging interaction among students, an engaging lecturer can foster a sense of community.

Also, senior's motivation and enjoyment of chair exercises can be significantly increased by involving family members. Exercise turns into a family activity that fosters camaraderie, creates enduring memories, and fortifies family ties.

1. **Creating a Family Fitness Routine:** Family members can schedule frequent workouts with their senior loved ones,

including fitness into their everyday schedule in a fun and interesting way. This shared commitment improves family ties and encourages healthy habits for future generations, whether it takes the form of a weekly chair exercise class or a workout at home.

2. **Making It Fun:** Formal exercise isn't the only way to involve the family. In addition to promoting physical activity, enjoyable events like dance parties, movement-based games, or just a stroll in the park can keep seniors engaged. The goal is to keep the atmosphere fun and lighthearted.

3. **Promoting Understanding and Support:** Family members can understand the importance of physical activity in maintaining independence and health by learning about the specific activities that help their senior loved ones. Seniors may find it easier to maintain their fitness routines as a result of this information, which may improve empathy and support.

4. **Creating Healthy Habits:** By including their families in exercise, seniors can serve as positive role models for coming generations. Family members may be inspired to live more active lives as a result of this interaction, promoting the general well-being of the family.

Even though social exercise has many benefits, some seniors may find it difficult to participate. Resolving these obstacles is essential to fostering a welcoming and encouraging environment.

1. **Transportation Problems:** Getting to community centers or group activities can be difficult for many seniors. Family members may help by providing transportation or setting up at-home workouts. Seniors may also be able to get transportation to classes through community initiatives.

2. **Health Issues:** Seniors may worry about their physical well-being and ability to engage in group exercise. It is crucial to make sure that trained instructors who can adapt exercises to various ability levels are teaching the classes. Seniors should consult their healthcare providers before starting a new exercise program, according to family members.

3. **Fear of Judgment:** In a group setting, seniors may feel self-conscious about their abilities. Creating a friendly work environment where everyone is encouraged, regardless of fitness level, is essential. Teachers and other participants' encouraging words may help ease these concerns.

4. **Lack of Knowledge:** Some elderly people might not be aware of the several options for family exercise or group sessions. Word-of-mouth from friends and family, flyers in neighborhood centers, and community outreach initiatives can all help people become more aware of the available possibilities.

For seniors over 70, adding social elements to chair exercise regimens is a great way to enhance their fitness experience. Seniors who take part in group classes and with their families can find motivation, responsibility, and a feeling of community. They may overcome interpersonal issues and enjoy their victories, which improves their general well-being and physical health. Seniors can make their fitness routines more enjoyable, long-lasting, and an essential part of their lives by forming social connections.

The Significance Of Warming Up

Any fitness program must include a warm-up, but it's especially important for seniors who do chair exercises. It entails progressively increasing blood flow, heart rate, and muscle temperature to prime the body for physical activity. In addition to enhancing performance, this pre-planning phase reduces the risk of injury. *We'll discuss the value of warming up, its benefits, and how to include it in your workout routine below:*

1. Advantages of the Physiology

- **Increased Oxygen Supply and Blood Flow:** Your heart rate increases as you warm up, which causes your body to pump more blood throughout it. The muscles receive more oxygen and nutrients from this increased blood flow, which is essential for optimal function. As muscles receive enough oxygen, they become more effective at producing energy, allowing for longer workouts. Since it guarantees that their bodies can withstand physical exertion safely, warming up is especially crucial for seniors who may have restricted circulation.

- **Increased Muscle Temperature:** Muscle flexibility and general function depend on increased muscle temperature, which is achieved through warming up. Joint range of motion is increased and stiffness is decreased by the increased flexibility of warmer muscles. Seniors, who may have stiffness due to age-related changes in their muscles and connective tissues, would particularly benefit from this. By increasing flexibility, warming up can enhance the comfort and efficacy of chair exercises for seniors.

2. Preventing Injuries

- **Reducing Muscular Strain:** Muscular strain is one of the most dangerous effects of working exercise without warming up. Pulls and tears are more likely to occur in cold muscles, which can be particularly harmful for older people. By using warm-ups to gradually increase the intensity of their activities, seniors can lower their risk of injury.

- **Joint Lubrication:** The production of synovial fluid, which lubricates joints, is encouraged by warming up. This is essential for maintaining joint function and health, particularly in elderly adults who may experience joint pain or arthritis. For chair workouts to be both safe and effective, joints that are well-lubricated can move more freely.

3. Mental Readiness

- **Psychological Readiness:** Warming up has a dual purpose in terms of the mind and body. It enables seniors to psychologically get ready for their workouts, focusing their attention on their health objectives rather than everyday distractions. Light physical activity can also lift your spirits, making exercise less intimidating and more enjoyable.

- **Creating a Routine:** You can create a persistent workout habit by incorporating a warm-up routine. It emphasizes the value of consistent exercise by telling the brain when it's time to engage in physical activity. A well-known warm-up can help seniors who lack the desire to start an exercise session more enthusiastically.

Warm-up Exercise Types

Moving different body parts while progressively increasing your reach, speed, or both is known as dynamic stretching. Arm circles, leg swings, and torso twists are a few examples. In addition to increasing flexibility, these actions prime the body for the specific motions needed for chair exercises.

1. **Soft Cardio:** The body can be warmed up with simple cardiovascular exercises like side bends, seated marching,

and soft toe taps. Without putting undue strain on the body, these exercises raise heart rate and blood circulation.

2. **Breathing Techniques:** Incorporating deep breathing exercises into the warm-up may aid in mental and physical relaxation. By increasing oxygen intake and lowering anxiety, deep breathing creates a positive atmosphere for the next session.

Suggestions for Senior Citizens

Seniors should warm up for five to ten minutes, increasing in intensity over time. The goal is to raise muscular temperature and heart rate without exerting too much effort. Start with gentle movements and work your way up to more vigorous ones.

Depending on each person's fitness level and any underlying medical issues, the warm-up should be modified. To prevent discomfort, seniors should pay attention to their bodies and make necessary modifications. People with restricted mobility may benefit greatly from seated warm-up exercises.

Seniors should make warming up a mandatory component of their exercise routine to reap the full advantages. As with any other workout, consistency is key to building general fitness, strength, and flexibility.

For seniors who do chair exercises in particular, warming up is a crucial step in getting the body ready for exercise. By increasing blood flow, warming up muscles, reducing the risk of injury, and fostering mental readiness, a proper warm-up can significantly increase the safety and effectiveness of a workout. For seniors to benefit from exercise safely and efficiently, warming up should be a crucial part of their fitness regimen.

In conclusion, it is impossible to overstate the significance of warming up; it is the foundation of a successful workout and lays the platform for improved mobility, independence, and health. Seniors who include a thorough warm-up routine can start their fitness adventures with joy and confidence, knowing they are taking important steps to safeguard their bodies while pursuing their health objectives.

Easy Warm-Up Exercises To Do While Seated

Warm-up activities are crucial for improving flexibility, preventing injuries, and preparing the body for more demanding physical activity. Warm-up exercises performed while seated can be a secure and efficient way for seniors, particularly those over 70, to get moving. By using this technique, people can benefit from exercising without running the danger of discomfort or falling. The seated warm-up exercises listed below target various muscle groups, increase blood flow and enhance overall health.

1. Marching while Seated

Time frame: two to three minutes

An efficient way to improve blood flow to the legs and get ready for other exercises is to march while seated.

Instructions:

1. Place your feet flat on the floor and sit up straight on a sturdy chair.
2. Raise one knee to your chest and raise the other arm to start the march.
3. Alternate sides steadily and slowly.

4. Breathe deeply and keep your posture correct.

2. Neck Rolls

Time frame: one to two minutes

Neck rolls are an essential warm-up for anyone who spends a lot of time sitting down since they help to release tension in the shoulders and neck.

Instructions:

1. With your shoulders relaxed and your back upright, take a comfortable seat.
2. Drop your right ear gently onto your right shoulder.
3. Allow your chin to sink into your chest as you slowly move your head forward.
4. Keep turning your head to the left until your left ear is close to your left shoulder.
5. Continue the sequence by going in the opposite direction.

3. Rolls of the Shoulders

Time frame: one to two minutes

By exercising the shoulder girdle, shoulder rolls improve the range of motion and lessen tension.

Instructions:

1. With your arms at your sides and your back straight, take a seat.
2. Lift your shoulders close to your ears and take a deep breath.
3. Roll your shoulders back and down as you release the breath.
4. After ten to fifteen repetitions, start moving your shoulders forward.

4. Arm Raises While Seated

Time frame: one to two minutes

Seated arm raises increase shoulder mobility and increase blood flow to the upper body.

1. With your feet flat on the ground, take a tall seat in your chair.
2. Raise both arms straight up and take a deep breath.
3. Lower your arms back to your sides and release the breath.
4. Pay attention to your breathing as you perform this action ten to fifteen times.

5. Torso twists

Time frame: one to two minutes

Torso twists increase core muscle flexibility and spinal mobility.

Instructions:

1. With your hands resting on your knees and your feet flat on the floor, sit up straight.
2. Take a deep breath and extend your back.
3. With your left hand supporting you on your right knee, carefully twist your torso to the right as you release your breath.
4. Return to the center after holding for a short while.
5. On the left side, repeat.
6. Twist each side five to ten times.

6. Rotations of the Wrist and Ankle

Time frame: two to three minutes

Rotations of the wrist and ankle are crucial for promoting mobility and warming up joints.

Instructions:

1. Rotate your wrists by extending one arm in front of you and pointing the palm down.
2. Before turning your wrist counterclockwise, rotate it clockwise for ten to fifteen seconds.
3. On the other wrist, repeat.
4. Rotate your ankle clockwise and counterclockwise for ten to fifteen seconds after raising one foot a little off the ground. Do the same with the other ankle.

7. Side bends when seated

Time frame: one to two minutes

By stretching the muscles on the sides of the body, seated side bends improve flexibility and ease tension.

Instructions:

1. Place your hands on your thighs and sit upright with your feet flat on the floor.
2. Take a breath and lift your right arm above your head.
3. Feel a stretch on your right side as you lean to the left and release your breath.
4. After a few seconds of holding, move back to the center.
5. On the other side, repeat.
6. Perform 5–10 reps on each side.

8. Heel Slides While Seated

Time frame: one to two minutes

Without putting undue strain on the joints, heel slides promote lower body movement and engage the legs.

Instructions:

1. With your back straight, take a seat at the edge of your chair.
2. Keeping the heel on the ground, extend one leg in front of you.
3. Bend your knee and gently bring your heel back nearer your body.
4. Do this ten to fifteen times on each leg.

9. Practice deep breathing

Time frame: two to three minutes

Any warm-up routine must include deep breathing since it improves oxygen flow and encourages calm.

Instructions:

1. With your hands on your knees, take a comfortable seat.
2. To expand your belly and fill your lungs, take a deep breath through your nose.
3. Pause and hold your breath.
4. Let your body relax as you release the breath slowly through your lips.
5. For five to ten breaths, repeat the technique.

Sitting warm-up exercises are a crucial component of fitness, particularly for older adults. These simple yet efficient workouts improve circulation and flexibility while getting the body ready for more demanding activities. Seniors can benefit from physical activity while putting their comfort and safety first by incorporating these seated warm-up exercises into their daily routines.

Techniques For Relaxing Breathing

Even though breathing is a vital aspect of life, many individuals undervalue its significance for both mental and physical well-being. Our breathing quickens and becomes shallow when we are stressed or anxious, which exacerbates tightness and uneasiness. On the other hand, employing specific breathing methods can promote calmness, lessen tension, and enhance overall health. To help elders and people of all ages relax and calm down, this section will examine several practical breathing techniques.

Understanding the significance of breath awareness is essential before delving into certain techniques. Being conscious of your breathing patterns and comprehending how they connect to your emotional and physical states is known as breath awareness. You can identify stressors and consciously switch to deeper, more calming breathing patterns by increasing your awareness of your breathing.

Breath awareness is a useful relaxation technique. *Here are some important things to think about:*

- By focusing on your breathing and being in the now, you might feel more grounded and less stressed and overwhelmed.

- You may be able to better regulate how you react to stress if you are aware of how your breathing fluctuates in response to certain emotions.
- In order to combat the fight-or-flight response brought on by stress, deep, steady breathing can trigger the body's relaxation response.

Relaxation Breathing Techniques

1. Belly Breathing, or Diaphragmatic Respiration

In order to improve oxygen absorption, diaphragmatic breathing—also referred to as belly breathing—involves drawing air deeply into the lungs. By promoting the parasympathetic nervous system, which calms the body, this method enhances relaxation.

Methods for Practice:

1. Choose a comfortable position to sit or lie in.
2. Two hands should be placed on your chest and abdomen, respectively.
3. Take a deep breath through your nose, allowing your chest to stay mostly stationary while your abdomen rises.
4. Feel your abdomen relax as you slowly release the breath through your lips.

5. Focus on the rise and fall of your abdomen as you repeat for a few minutes.

2. 4-7-8 Inhaling

The 4-7-8 breathing technique was created by Dr. Andrew Weil with the goal of promoting relaxation and reducing anxiety. For accurate counts, this method involves taking a deep breath, holding it, and then letting it out.

Methods for Practice:

1. Begin by finding a comfortable posture to sit or sleep.
2. For four counts, close your eyes and take a deep breath through your nostrils.
3. For the count of seven, hold your breath.
4. For a count of eight, slowly and completely exhale through your mouth.
5. For four complete breaths, repeat this cycle, increasing the number of repetitions as you become more at ease.

3. Square Breathing, or Box Breathing

Sports and military personnel employ box breathing, a straightforward yet effective technique, to increase focus and lower stress. This method creates a "box" rhythm by inhaling, holding, exhaling, and holding the breath for equal counts.

Methods for Practice:

1. Maintain a straight back when sitting comfortably.
2. Take a deep breath through your nose for four counts.
3. For four counts, hold your breath.
4. Take a slow, four-count breath out of your mouth.
5. For another count of four, hold your breath.
6. For a few minutes, repeat this cycle while paying attention to your breathing rhythm.

4. Alternate Nostril Breathing, or Nadi Shodhana

Alternating nostril breathing, or nadi shodhana, is a yoga technique for balancing the body's energy and promoting mental peace. This exercise can help you feel less stressed and think more clearly.

Methods for Practice:

1. Maintain a straight spine when sitting comfortably.
2. Seal your right nostril with your thumb.
3. Take a deep breath through your left nostril.
4. Using your right ring finger, close your left nostril, then open your right nostril.
5. Breathe out through your right nostril.
6. Close your right nostril with your thumb after taking a big breath.
7. Breathe through your left nostril after releasing it.
8. For several minutes, keep doing this while focusing on your breathing sensations.

5. Breathing Visualization

By stimulating your imagination, visualization combined with breathing might help you relax. With this method, you can concentrate on your breathing while visualizing a calm scene.

Methods for Practice:

1. Find a position that feels comfortable, then close your eyes.
2. Breathe deeply a few times to find your core.
3. Imagine a soothing hue or setting (such as a serene beach or forest) when you take a breath.

4. Imagine releasing stress and tension into the atmosphere as you exhale.
5. Keep doing this for a few minutes so that you can fully immerse yourself in the visualization.

There are several advantages to using different breathing techniques for relaxation and general health, such as:

- **Decreased Anxiety and Stress:** Deep, slow breathing triggers the parasympathetic nervous system, which lowers anxiety and cortisol levels.
- **Increased Concentration and Focus:** By using mindful breathing techniques, you can increase your concentration and mental clarity, which will make it easier for you to complete activities.
- **Improved Sleep Quality:** You can fall and stay asleep more easily if you incorporate breathing techniques into your nightly routine.
- **Better Physical Health:** Deep breathing promotes oxygen flow throughout the body, which is good for the heart and vitality in general.

Include these breathing exercises in your daily practice to get the most out of them:

- **Practice in the Morning:** To create a positive atmosphere, start each day with a few minutes of deep breathing.
- **Use in Stressful Situations:** Take a moment to practice one of the breathing techniques to help you regain control when you're feeling overburdened or pressured.
- **Establish a Relaxation Routine:** Schedule time each day for relaxation, incorporating breathing exercises with other calming pursuits like meditation or gentle stretching.

Breathing techniques are a powerful tool for enhancing general well-being, lowering stress, and encouraging relaxation. By incorporating these techniques into your everyday routine, you may strengthen your resilience and sense of calm, which will make it easier for you to deal with life's challenges. Finding a strategy that works for you and incorporating it into your wellness routine is crucial, regardless of whether you choose to employ diaphragmatic breathing, 4-7-8 breathing, box breathing, or another method.

CHAPTER 3: SIMPLE CHAIR EXERCISES FOR SENIORS

For Physical Strength

1. Seated Toe Taps

Instructions:

1. Sit in a chair with your feet flat on the floor.
2. Lift your right foot and tap your toes against the floor before you, then return to the starting position.
3. Repeat with the left foot, alternating sides.

Benefits:

1. Strengthens the lower legs and enhances ankle flexibility.
2. Controlled motions help to improve coordination and balance.
3. Strengthens the lower leg muscles, which are required for daily activities like walking.

2. Seated Eagle Pose

Instructions:

1. Sit straight on your chair, feet level on the ground.
2. Cross your arms in front of you, one below the other.
3. Bend your elbows and bring your hands together. Hold this position for a few breaths.
4. Release and repeat on the other side.

Benefits:

1. Includes greater upper-body flexibility and shoulder range of motion.
2. Reduces strain in the upper back.
3. Increases focus and concentration through mindful movement.

3. Seated Mountain Pose

Instructions:

1. Sit upright on a chair, feet flat on the floor and hands resting on knees.
2. Take a deep inhalation while holding your arms high and palms facing each other.

3. Hold the pose for a few breaths and feel the stretch in your spine.
4. Exhale, then lower your arms to your knees.

Benefits:

1. Enhances core strength and posture stability.
2. Increases awareness of breathing and body alignment.
3. Focused breathing and stretching can assist in alleviating anxiety.

4. Seated Banded Chest Press

Instructions:

1. Sit erect in a sturdy chair, feet level with the ground and back straight.
2. Place a resistance band over your back and fasten it to the back of the chair.
3. Hold the band handles at shoulder height, palms facing front, and elbows bent 90 degrees.
4. Exhale and push the grips forward, fully extending your arms and keeping your elbows slightly bent.
5. Pause at the end of the movement, inhale, and return to the starting position with control.

1. Increases upper-body strength by strengthening the pectoral, deltoids, and triceps muscles.
2. Improves shoulder stability and functional mobility.
3. Improves posture by strengthening the chest and shoulder muscles.

5. Seated Bicep Curls

Instructions:

1. Sit on a chair with a dumbbell in each hand, arms at your sides, and palms facing forward.
2. Exhale as you curl the weights up to your shoulders, keeping your elbows close to your body.
3. Squeeze your biceps at the peak of the movement, then inhale as you lower the weights back to their starting position.

Benefits:

1. Isolates and develops the biceps, which improves arm strength and tone.
2. Increases grip strength, which is necessary for regular tasks.

3. Enhances functional movements, making tasks like lifting goods easier.

6. Seated Shoulder Press

Instructions:

1. Sit on an upright chair with a dumbbell in each hand at shoulder level, palms facing forward.
2. Exhale and press the dumbbells overhead until your arms are fully extended.
3. Lower the weights to shoulder height while breathing, and maintain control throughout the exercise.

Benefits:

1. Increases shoulder muscular strength, allowing for increased overhead mobility.
2. Improves shoulder joint stability and lowers the risk of injury.
3. Promotes proper posture and upper-body strength.

7. Seated Side Stretch

Instructions:

1. Sit tall in a chair, feet flat on the ground.
2. Raise your right arm overhead and bend to the left until you feel a stretch along your right side.
3. Pause for a few breaths before returning to the middle and continuing on the other side.

Benefits:

1. Improves spinal and torso flexibility.
2. Helps to reduce tension in the sides and lower back.
3. Improves breathing patterns by extending the chest and rib cage.

8. Modified Chair Squats

Instructions:

1. Sit on the edge of a sturdy chair, feet hip-width apart, flat on the floor.
2. Lean slightly forward and rise from your chair, utilizing your core and leg muscles.
3. Carefully lower yourself back into your chair.

1. Increases lower-body strength, especially with the quadriceps, hamstrings, and glutes.
2. Increases functional mobility, making it easier to stand from a sitting position.
3. Promotes balance and stability.

For Heart Health

1. Seated Forward Bent

Instructions:

1. Sit erect in a chair with your feet flat on the floor.
2. Inhale and then raise your arms high.
3. Exhale as you lean forward at the hips and lower your hands to the floor or rest them on your legs.
4. Hold for a few breaths, letting your back lengthen and your head hang low.
5. Inhale to return to an upright position.

Benefits:

1. Improves spine and hamstring flexibility.
2. Improves circulation throughout the body.
3. Reduces stress and promotes relaxation.

2. Foot-to-Seat Pose

Instructions:

1. Sit in a sturdy chair with a straight back and level feet.
2. Lift your right foot and place it on your left thigh.
3. Hold your back straight and gently press down on your right knee to increase the stretch.
4. Hold for a few breaths, then switch legs.

Benefits:

1. Increases hip and thigh flexibility.
2. Increases blood flow to the legs, potentially helping to alleviate stiffness.
3. Improves posture by opening the hips.

3. Palm Tree Pose

Instructions:

1. Sit upright in a chair, feet flat on the floor.
2. Inhale and raise your arms, interlocking your fingers.
3. Reach up to the ceiling and lengthen your spine.
4. Hold for a few breaths, then lower your arms.

1. Enhances upper-body strength and flexibility.
2. Encourages deep breathing, which benefits heart health.
3. Improves focus and balance, leading to increased stability.

4. Triangle Position

Instructions:

1. Sit in a chair with your right leg extended to the side and your foot flat on the ground.
2. Raise your left arm straight up and reach over your right leg for a side stretch.
3. Hold for a few breaths, then switch sides.

Benefits:

1. Improves side-body flexibility and core strength.
2. Increases flexibility in the legs and hips, which improves mobility.
3. Encourages deep breathing, which may help lower blood pressure.

5. Seated Leg Stretches

Instructions:

1. Sit on the edge of your chair, feet flat on the floor.
2. Stretch your right leg straight in front of you, flexing your foot.
3. Hold for a few seconds until you feel the stretch in your calf and hamstring.
4. Lower your leg, then switch to your left leg.

Benefits:

1. Increases flexibility in the hamstrings and calves.
2. Increases circulation in the legs, which is beneficial to heart health.
3. Helps to reduce muscle tension.

6. Calf Stretches

Instructions:

1. Sit with your back straight and your feet flat on the ground.
2. Extend one leg forward, heel on the ground, toes pointed upwards.
3. Lean slightly forward and feel the stretch in your calf.

4. Hold for a few breaths, then switch legs.

Benefits:

1. Increases calves' flexibility and suppleness.
2. Improves circulation, which is essential for heart health.
3. It helps to relieve cramps and stiffness in the lower legs.

7. Chair Squat

Instructions:

1. Sit at the edge of the chair, feet hip-width apart.
2. Lean slightly forward and rise from the chair with your legs, keeping your back straight.
3. To sit without using your hands, gently lower yourself back down.
4. Repeat several times.

Benefits:

1. Improves leg strength and balance.
2. Increased physical activity helps to improve heart health.
3. Improves coordination and steadiness.

8. Seated Knee to Chest Pose

Instructions:

1. Sit straight in your chair, feet level with the ground.
2. Bring one knee up to your chest and hold it in both hands.
3. Hold for a few breaths before lowering and swapping legs.

Benefits:

Reduces stiffness in the lower back and hips.
Improves the circulation in the lower body.
Promotes relaxation and reduces tension.

For Wheelchair Patients

1. Seated Chest Expansions

Instructions:

1. Sit upright in your wheelchair, back straight.
2. Hold a resistance band or keep your arms extended in front of you at shoulder height.
3. Slowly pull your arms outward, stretching the band or spreading your arms to the sides, elbows slightly bent.
4. Squeeze your shoulder blades together and extend your chest.
5. Maintain the position for a few seconds before returning to the starting position.
6. Repeat 10–15 times.

Benefits:

1. Improves upper-body strength and flexibility.
2. Activates the upper back and chest muscles, hence improving posture and spinal alignment.
3. Increases lung capacity and breathing efficiency.

2. Seated Side Arm Stretches

Instructions:

1. Sit upright in your wheelchair, feet flat on the floor or footrests.
2. Raise one arm overhead and extend to the opposite side.
3. Hold the stretch for 15-30 seconds, feeling it down your side.
4. Return to the starting position, then repeat on the opposing side.
5. Repeat 5 to 10 times, switching sides.

Benefits:

1. Increases lateral flexibility and movement in the torso.
2. Helps to relieve tension in the shoulders and neck.
3. Encourages deep breathing for relaxation and mental clarity.

3. Seated Dive Stretches

Instructions:

1. Sit upright in your wheelchair, feet flat on the ground.
2. Lean forward and extend your arms overhead, aiming to reach your toes or as far as you are comfortable.
3. Hold the pose for a few seconds and breathe deeply.
4. Gradually return to the upright position.
5. Repeat 5–10 times.

Benefits:

1. Improves overall flexibility and range of motion.
2. Controlled movement encourages relaxation and stress alleviation.

4. Seated Raised Arm Circles

Instructions:

1. Sit upright in your wheelchair, feet flat on the floor.
2. Extend your arms to the sides at shoulder height.
3. Begin by drawing little circles with your arms and progressively increase the size of each circle.

4. Draw 10 circles in one direction, then switch to the opposite direction.
5. Ensure that your core is engaged throughout the action.

Benefits:

1. Increases shoulder mobility and stability.
2. Improves circulation in the arms and upper body.
3. It helps to relieve stiffness and stress in the shoulder joints.

5. Seated Overhead Punches

Instructions:

1. Sit upright with your feet firmly on the ground.
2. Raise your right arm overhead, as if to punch upward.
3. Return to the starting position and repeat with the left arm.
4. Repeat 10-15 times, alternating between the arms.

Benefits:

1. Strengthens the shoulders, arms, and upper chest.
2. Improves coordination and rhythm.
3. Improves cardiovascular health by raising the heart rate during exercise.

6. Seated Hip Stretches

Instructions:

1. Sit upright in your wheelchair, back straight.
2. Place one ankle on the other knee.
3. Gently press down on the elevated knee to lengthen the stretch.
4. Hold the stretch for 15 to 30 seconds before switching legs.
5. Repeat 5–10 stretches on each side.

Benefits:

1. Enhances hip flexibility.
2. It reduces stress and pain in the lower body.
3. Improves blood circulation in the lower extremities.

7. Seated Leg Stretches

Instructions:

1. Sit upright with your back straight and your feet level on the floor.
2. Extend one leg straight in front of you and keep it parallel to the ground.

3. Stay in this position for a few seconds before lowering your leg back down.
4. Repeat with the opposing leg.
5. Perform 5–10 repetitions per leg.

Benefits:

1. Improves leg strength and mobility.
2. Stretches the hamstrings and calves.
3. Enhances lower-body coordination and stability.

8. Seated Twist

Instructions:

1. Sit upright in your wheelchair, feet flat.
2. Swivel your torso to the right while holding the wheelchair's back with your right hand.
3. Hold the position for 15-30 seconds, feeling the stretch in your back.
4. Return to the center and repeat on the left side.
5. Repeat 5 to 10 times, switching sides.

Benefits:

1. Increases spinal flexibility and mobility.
2. Reduces stress in the back and shoulders.
3. Increases core stability and strength.

For Weight Loss

1. Seated Pigeon Pose

Instructions:

1. Sit tall in your chair, right ankle on your left knee.
2. Inhale to lengthen your spine, then exhale as you softly lean forward, keeping your back straight.
3. Hold the stance for a few breaths while feeling the stretch in your hip.
4. Switch sides and repeat.

Benefits:

1. Opens the hips, which relieves tension and discomfort.
2. Enhances lower-body flexibility.
3. Reduces tension and anxiety.

2. Chair's Extended Side Angle

Instructions:

1. Sit on the edge of your chair, feet firmly planted on the ground.
2. Perform a side stretch by extending your right arm over you and leaning to the left.
3. Use your left hand to support your left knee.
4. Hold for a few breaths, feeling the stretch in your side body.
5. Switch sides and repeat.

Benefits:

1. Improves flexibility in the spine and side body.
2. It strengthens the core and the obliques.
3. Enhances balance and coordination.

3. Seated Leg Raises

Instructions:

1. Sit up straight with your back against the chair.
2. Extend your right leg straight ahead of you, keeping it parallel to the ground.

3. Hold for a few seconds to activate your core, then drop it back down.
4. Repeat 10–15 times, then switch to your left leg.

Benefits:

1. Strengthens the hip flexors and quadriceps, boosting muscle tone.
2. Improves core stability and balance.
3. Helps to burn calories and encourages weight loss.

4. Seated Cat-Cow

Instructions:

1. Sit up straight with your feet flat on the floor and your hands on your knees.
2. Inhale, arch your back and gaze up (Cow Pose).
3. Exhale, curve your back and tuck your chin toward your chest (Cat Pose).
4. Continue to alternate between these two positions for 5-10 breaths.

Benefits:

1. Enhances spinal flexibility and posture.
2. Reduces stress in the back and neck.
3. Encourages relaxation and stress reduction.

5. Seated Warrior II

Instructions:

1. Sit upright on your chair, feet flat on the floor.
2. Extend your right leg to the side, maintaining it straight, and bend your left knee.
3. Raise your arms parallel to the floor and examine your right fingertips.
4. Pause for a few breaths before swapping sides.

Benefits:

1. Improves lower-body strength and stability.
2. Improves concentration and mental focus.
3. Opens the hips and chest, improving overall flexibility.

6. Seated Sun Salutation

Instructions:

1. Sit tall with your hands at your heart's center.
2. Inhale while raising your arms upward and stretching your spine.
3. Exhale, then fold into a forward bend.
4. Inhale, lift back to the starting position and repeat the cycle several times.

Benefits:

1. Increases energy levels in both the body and mind.
2. Improves general flexibility and circulation.
3. Breathing encourages mindfulness and relaxation.

7. Seated Forward Fold Pose (Paschimottanasana)

Instructions:

1. Sit on the edge of a sturdy chair, feet level with the floor and hip-width apart.
2. Inhale deeply and lift your arms high to lengthen your spine.

3. Exhale, then fold forward, bending at the hips and reaching for your feet, shins, or ankles.
4. Lean forward with your spine long to avoid rounding your back.
5. Hold the pose for a few breaths, feeling the stretch in your hamstrings and back.
6. To release, slowly return to an upright position.

Benefits:

1. Boosts flexibility by stretching the spine, hamstrings, and shoulders.
2. Helps to alleviate anxiety and stress, which improves overall mental health.
3. Improves digestion and alleviates insomnia symptoms.

8. Seated Twist

Instructions:

1. Sit erect in a chair with your feet flat on the floor.
2. Inhale to lengthen your spine, then exhale and twist your torso to the right, keeping your left hand on your knee and your right hand behind you on the chair.
3. Maintain the twist for a few breaths, intensifying with each exhale.

4. Inhale to return to the center, then repeat on the left side.

Benefits:

1. Improves spinal mobility and flexibility.
2. Massages the internal organs, encouraging digestion.
3. Helps to relieve tension in the back and shoulders.

To Improve Posture

1. Seated Reverse Warrior

Instructions:

1. Sit on the edge of a chair, legs spread wide.
2. Inhale, then stretch one arm overhead, leaning toward the opposite leg.
3. Hold the position for 15-30 seconds, keeping your body stretched and your neck relaxed.
4. Switch sides and repeat.

Benefits:

1. Increases leg strength and side-body flexibility.
2. Improves general balance and coordination.
3. Deep, deliberate breathing helps to increase lung capacity.

2. Seated Chest Opener

Instructions:

1. Sit at the edge of the chair, with your feet flat on the ground.
2. Inhale as you raise your arms to the sides and clasp your hands behind your back.
3. Exhale and gently draw your shoulder blades together to elevate your chest.
4. Hold for 15-30 seconds, inhaling deeply.

Benefits:

1. Opening the chest and improving posture.
2. Relieves stiffness in the shoulders and upper back.
3. Improves breathing by expanding the chest area.

3. Seated High Alternate Lean

Instructions:

1. Sit on the chair's edge, feet on the floor.
2. Inhale while holding both arms up, then exhale while leaning slightly to one side.

3. Hold for 15-30 seconds before moving back to the center and switching sides.

Benefits:

1. Increases lateral flexibility and stretches the sides of the torso.
2. It promotes proper posture by stretching the spine.
3. Increases circulation throughout the body.

4. Seated Camel Pose

Instructions:

1. Sit tall on the edge of a sturdy chair, feet level with the floor and shoulder width apart.
2. Inhale deeply, raising your chest and bringing your shoulders back.
3. Exhale as you gently arch your back and reach for your heels or the chair behind you.
4. Keep your neck flexible and don't extend your head too far back.
5. Hold for 15-30 seconds, inhaling deeply.

1. Stretching the front body and increasing spinal flexibility.
2. Strengthens the back muscles, which improves posture.
3. Increases lung capacity and enhances respiratory function.

5. Seated Happy Baby Pose

Instructions:

1. Sit on the edge of a chair, with your feet flat on the floor.
2. Bend your knees and lift your feet off the ground, holding your knees in your hands.
3. Pull your knees softly toward your armpits while keeping your back straight.
4. Hold the pose for 15-30 seconds, inhaling deeply.

Benefits:

1. Reduces lower back tension and increases hip mobility.
2. Increases flexibility in the groin and hip areas.
3. Promotes relaxation and reduces tension.

6. Extended Triangle Stance

Instructions:

1. Sit with legs apart and feet flexed.
2. Inhale, raise your arms and exhale while bending toward one leg, hand on the thigh, or foot.
3. Extend the second arm straight up and keep your torso open.
4. Hold for 15-30 seconds, then switch sides.

Benefits:

1. Improves balance and coordination.
2. Strengthens the legs and stretches the sides of the body.
3. Increases flexibility and reduces spinal tension.

7. Chair Spinal Twist

Instructions:

1. Sit erect on your chair, feet level on the ground.
2. Inhale to lengthen your spine, then exhale and twist your torso to one side, using the backrest as support.
3. Hold for 15-30 seconds, then switch sides.

1. Increases spinal flexibility and mobility.
2. Reduces lower back pain by encouraging appropriate alignment.
3. Gentle belly massage improves digestion.

For Flexibility, Mobility, And Balance

1. Seated Sage 3 Pose

Instructions:

1. Sit upright in your chair and extend one leg straight in front.
2. Maintain a long spine by stretching your hands towards the foot of your extended leg.
3. Hold for 30 seconds, then switch sides.

Benefits:

1. Greater hamstring and lower back length.
2. Improves spinal flexibility.
3. Improves posture and reduces stiffness.

2. Seated wide-legged. Forward Fold

Instructions:

1. Sit on the edge of the chair, feet apart.
2. Inhale to lengthen your spine, then exhale and bend forward from the hips.
3. Rest your hands on the floor or your thighs, keeping your back flat.

4. Hold for 30-60 seconds.

Benefits:

1. Stretches the inner thighs and lower back.
2. Improves hip mobility.
3. Reduces lower-body tension, promoting relaxation.

3. Seated Knee-to-Chest Pose

Instructions:

1. Sit tall in your chair, feet flat on the floor.
2. Bring one knee to your chest and hold it in both hands.
3. Gently bring your knee closer while keeping your back straight.
4. Hold for 20-30 seconds, then switch legs.

Benefits:

1. Improves the lower back and hip flexors.
2. Improves hip mobility.
3. Reduces tension in the lower spine.

4. King Arthur's Pose

Instructions:

1. Sit tall in your chair, feet flat on the floor.
2. Extend one leg straight out in front, heel on the ground.
3. Tilt forward slowly from the hips, reaching for your extended foot while keeping your back flat.
4. Hold the stretch for 20-30 seconds, then switch sides.

Benefits:

1. Increases hamstring flexibility.
2. Strengthens the lower back.
3. Improves posture and reduces muscle stress in the legs.

5. Seated Tree Pose

Instructions:

1. Sit upright on your chair, feet flat on the floor.
2. Lift your right foot and place its sole against the inner left thigh or calf.
3. Raise your arms, and palms together.
4. Hold for 20-30 seconds, then switch legs.

Benefits:

1. Improves balance and coordination.
2. It develops the core and leg muscles.
3. Improves concentration and physical awareness.

6. Seated Bound Angle Pose

Instructions:

1. Sit at the edge of the chair, back straight.
2. Bring the soles of your feet together and gradually lower your knees to the side.
3. Hold your feet with your hands and keep a long spine.
4. Maintain the pose for 30 seconds to 1 minute.

Benefits:

1. Improves the hips, inner thighs, and groin.
2. Increases hip flexibility.
3. Improves circulation throughout the lower body.

7. Extended Side Angle Pose

Instructions:

1. Sit erect, feet wide apart and toes pointed forward.
2. Raise your right arm to the sky, then rest your left elbow on your left thigh.
3. Stretch to the side, keeping your chest open.
4. Hold for 20-30 seconds, then switch sides.

Benefits:

1. Strengthens the obliques and legs.
2. Improves hip and spinal flexibility.
3. Enhances balance and stability.

8. Seated Tummy Twists

Instructions:

1. Sit upright, feet flat on the floor.
2. Twist your torso to the right while gripping the side of the chair with your hands.
3. Maintain a straight spine as you deepen the twist with each exhalation.
4. Hold for 20-30 seconds, then switch sides.

1. Increases spine flexibility.
2. Improves digestion and reduces bloating.
3. Strengthens the core muscles.

CHAPTER 4: MAINTAINING MOTIVATION AND OVERCOMING OBSTACLES

Typical Exercise Barriers And How To Overcome Them

For seniors who wish to preserve or improve their health, exercise offers several mental, emotional, and physical advantages. Even with the proven advantages, many elderly people have significant barriers to engaging in regular physical activity. Remaining active and leading a healthier, more independent lifestyle depends on identifying and overcoming these obstacles. *We'll examine some common obstacles to senior fitness below and provide workable ways to get beyond them:*

1. Physical Restrictions

Physical limitations like arthritis, joint pain, and decreased movement are common as people age. Because of these challenges, traditional forms of exercise may seem daunting, leading to anxiety about injury or discomfort. Starting a fitness regimen can be intimidating for seniors who are currently managing chronic illnesses.

How to Get Past Physical Restrictions

1. Walking, swimming, and chair exercises are all beneficial low-impact activities for seniors. These workouts improve strength and flexibility while reducing joint stress. For instance, chair workouts reduce the chance of injury by enabling users to concentrate on several muscle groups while still seated.

2. A lot of exercises can be modified to accommodate certain physical limitations. For example, using a chair to provide support during exercises like lunges or squats might reduce their intensity without sacrificing their advantages. For people with severe arthritis, mild range-of-motion exercises can help reduce stiffness and enhance mobility.

3. Seniors should speak with their physical therapist or healthcare provider before beginning any new fitness regimen to see whether exercises are suitable for their medical condition.

2. Fear of Falls or Injuries

Among elderly people, fear of injury—especially falls—is a major worry. Activities requiring balance or coordination, such as walking on uneven terrain, standing exercises, or weight-bearing activities, may be avoided by people who are terrified of falling. This anxiety often results in inactivity, which can impair physical well-being and raise the risk of falls due to weakened muscles.

How to Deal with Injury Fear:

1. By incorporating strength and balance training into your training regimen, you can significantly reduce your risk of falling. Seniors who are worried about their balance can benefit greatly from chair exercises. Stability is increased by strengthening the legs and core with exercises like seated leg lifts and seated marches.

2. To help elders stay balanced and prevent falls during exercise, they can use support equipment like chairs, railings, or even resistance bands. For instance, standing exercises can be made more stable by using a chair.

3. It's important to start cautiously and build your confidence over time. Start with easy, low-intensity exercises and work

your way up to more difficult ones as your strength and balance get better. As their skills grow, elders can feel less fearful of damage and more secure thanks to this gradual approach.

3. Insufficient Drive

Many people find it difficult to stay motivated to work out. Seniors may lack motivation because of emotions of tiredness, past failures, or a lack of quick results. It is easy to become inactive without a well-thought-out plan or outside assistance.

How to Handle Low Motivation:

1. Maintaining motivation requires setting tiny, achievable goals. Achievable goals that give you a sense of accomplishment include "walking for 10 minutes a day" and "doing three chair exercises each week." These goals may be modified when progress is made in order to maintain the feeling of challenge and development.

2. Staying motivated requires consistency. A consistent exercise regimen, such as designating specific days and times for exercise, can help seniors make exercise a part of their everyday routine. This makes it easier to maintain

momentum by reducing the mental effort needed to start a session.

3. Working out in a group setting or with a friend or relative can improve the experience and encourage responsibility. Sharing your fitness journey with others will help you stay on track because social interaction is a strong motivator. Senior-friendly fitness programs that blend social contact with health are available in many locations, either in-person or online.

4. Restricted Availability of Exercise Equipment and Facilities

Not everyone has access to specialized exercise equipment, gyms, or swimming pools. Seniors may be discouraged from beginning or maintaining a fitness routine due to this lack of availability, particularly if they feel that they need certain equipment in order to exercise.

How to Deal with Restricted Access:

1. With minimal or no equipment, a variety of great workouts may be done in the convenience of one's own house. Stretching exercises, chair workouts, and bodyweight exercises are all excellent examples of activities that call for minimal space and equipment. To perform a variety of

strengthening and mobility exercises, a sturdy chair and resistance bands are sufficient.

2. There are several websites that offer low-cost or free exercise programs designed for senior citizens. These can be accessed via a smartphone, tablet, or computer, enabling elders to work out under supervision at home. Seek out programs created especially for senior citizens, with adjustments made to account for different skill levels.

3. Senior exercise classes are offered for free or at a reduced cost by a number of community centers, senior centers, and recreation centers in the area. These programs usually include swimming, walking, or group classes, which provide an organized environment for maintaining an active lifestyle.

5. Exhaustion and Low Energy

Seniors often struggle with fatigue, particularly those who have long-term conditions like diabetes or heart disease. This lack of energy could make working out seem overwhelming or difficult. Nonetheless, regular exercise has been shown to gradually increase energy levels, making it a crucial part of managing fatigue.

How to Handle Exhaustion:

1. It's important to start with brief, manageable activity sessions for seniors who are struggling with fatigue. As your energy levels improve, progressively increase the amount of time you spend moving, starting with simply 5–10 minutes of light activities like seated exercises or leisurely walking.

2. Getting proper rest in between workouts is just as important as maintaining consistency. Elderly people can manage their exhaustion while being active by taking rest days, which give their bodies time to recover and rejuvenate.

3. Certain times of the day give some people extra energy. Seniors should work out in the morning, afternoon, or evening when they are most energetic. This could make the workout more enjoyable and less taxing.

6. Persistent Medical Conditions

Chronic conditions like diabetes, heart disease, or lung problems might make exercise seem risky or challenging. Seniors may not exercise at all since they don't know what kinds of physical activities are safe for their condition.

How to Handle Long-Term Medical Issues:

1. It is important to see a physician before starting any fitness program, especially for elderly patients who have chronic illnesses. Considering any limitations or risks to the person's health, a medical professional can suggest particular activities that are both beneficial and safe.

2. Regular exercise is crucial for managing symptoms and maintaining general health, even for elderly people with chronic illnesses. Stretching, walking, and chair yoga are examples of low-intensity exercises that can help increase cardiovascular health, strength, and flexibility without placing an excessive amount of strain on the body.

By removing these common obstacles, seniors can improve their mobility, health, and quality of life by incorporating regular exercise into their lives. A more active and fulfilling life can result from overcoming these obstacles, whether via adjustments, social support, or customized routines.

Advice On How To Stay Accountable And Motivated

It can occasionally be challenging to stay accountable and motivated while following a fitness regimen, particularly for seniors who engage in chair exercises. It might be challenging to stay active due to obstacles in life, health issues, or just a lack of energy. However, staying on track with your fitness goals is both achievable and fulfilling if you have the right attitude and strategies. Let's examine some doable strategies for helping seniors maintain their motivation and responsibility while they use chair exercises to improve their health.

1. Establish attainable and unambiguous goals

One of the best ways to keep yourself motivated is to set clear, achievable goals. Establishing specific objectives for your fitness journey gives you focus and direction. These goals ought to be doable and appropriate for your level of fitness. For instance, aim for 15 minutes of action three times a week if you're just starting off with chair exercises. Increase the length or intensity gradually as you advance.

It's important to refrain from setting unrealistic goals since they could cause harm or discontent. Divide lofty goals into more manageable benchmarks. Reaching one of these goals gives

you a sense of accomplishment and motivates you to keep
going.

2. Monitor your progress

Monitoring your progress is essential to holding yourself
responsible. You get a sense of success and are inspired to keep
going when you can see the results of your hard work. A great
approach to documenting your workouts is to keep a fitness
notebook, where you may note the exercises you performed,
your feelings during the session, and any improvements in your
strength, flexibility, or endurance.

Digital fitness monitors are also helpful to some elderly people.
These gadgets can monitor your heart rate while exercising, as
well as your activity and caloric expenditure. Maintaining a
record of your progress, whether through a conventional
notebook or a technological method, can serve as a strong
motivator.

3. Establish a routine

Creating a regular exercise regimen is essential to creating
enduring habits. Because exercise is already scheduled into
your calendar, routine eliminates the need to decide whether
to do it each day. As with any other appointment, it's a good

idea to plan your chair workouts for specific days and times and to keep to them.

For instance, you may schedule your workouts for just after breakfast on Mondays, Wednesdays, and Fridays. A timetable can give your week structure and a sense of routine, which can make it simpler to follow, especially on days when you're not feeling very motivated. Your exercise routine will eventually become a natural part of your everyday life if you are consistent.

4. Have fun

Working out doesn't have to be difficult. Making your chair training routine enjoyable is one way to stay motivated. This can be achieved by combining your favorite activities or by making small changes to keep things interesting. For instance, play your favorite music or audiobook while working out. You feel more engaged and enthusiastic about your workout when you listen to music, which has a significant impact on your mood and energy levels.

You could also try working out in a different environment. Do your chair exercises outside on a sunny day if at all possible. A change of scenery and some fresh air can keep you inspired and make you value the experience more. Finding ways to inject enjoyment and excitement into your exercise routine could be crucial to maintaining motivation over time.

5. Ask friends and family for help

The assistance of others can greatly ease the burden of staying accountable. When you don't feel like working out, involving friends, family, or even a workout partner can help you stay inspired and motivated. Either in person or virtually through a video call, you can ask a friend or relative to join you in your chair exercises. Working out with others can make it more enjoyable and less like a one-off effort by turning it into a social event.

Talking to a loved one about your health goals may also help you maintain accountability. They can give you encouraging feedback and conduct routine check-ins to see how your workouts are going. You may be more motivated to be consistent if you know that someone else is working hard for your success.

6. Reward yourself

Another good strategy for maintaining motivation is rewarding oneself for reaching objectives or finishing exercises. These rewards don't have to be expensive; they can be as simple as spending time on a hobby you enjoy or enjoying your favorite snack. Making a link between your achievements and positive experiences is the goal.

For instance, treat yourself to a relaxing bath or a viewing of your preferred television program after a week of regular chair exercises. These modest incentives can generate a positive feedback loop, reinforcing your dedication to your exercise practice. Celebrating your victory, no matter how modest, can help you stay happy and motivated.

7. Focus on the benefits

It's easy to lose sight of why you started exercising in the first place, especially on days when you're not feeling particularly energetic or inspired. To combat this, remind yourself on a regular basis of the benefits of chair exercises. Whether it's enhancing your mobility, flexibility, or mental wellness, focusing on the favorable consequences helps renew your excitement.

Keep a list of your reasons for exercising somewhere visible, such as on your refrigerator or bathroom mirror. This visual reminder will serve as a daily nudge, keeping you focused on your "why" and maintaining a good attitude toward your fitness path.

8. Adapt to adversities

Maintaining a fitness routine could be challenging at times due to life's responsibilities. Challenges are inescapable, whether they are connected to health, a tight schedule, or a lack of energy. Learning to adjust is vital for maintaining motivation and accountable. If you skip a day or two of exercise, don't be too hard on yourself; simply start up where you left off.

Flexibility is crucial, particularly as you traverse the ups and downs of life. If you aren't feeling up to your typical routine, you can adjust the exercises or do a shorter session. The crucial thing is to keep moving, even if at a reduced rate. You can overcome short-term obstacles and keep up your pace if you are adaptive.

9. Join an exercise club for seniors

Participating in an online or in-person senior exercise class or club can provide a sense of camaraderie and help you stay on schedule. For many seniors, belonging to a group keeps them engaged and motivated. Social interaction, support, and a common goal are all made possible in group situations. It is simpler to show up and put in the work when you are aware that others are joining you.

These days, online platforms offer a variety of fitness programs tailored to senior citizens, including chair workouts. By offering guidance and discipline, these sessions help you remain on course and meet others who share your fitness objectives.

10. Imagine yourself successful

One of the most important tools for maintaining motivation is visualization. Take a few moments every day to see yourself reaching your fitness goals, whether they involve losing weight, getting stronger, or regaining your mobility. When you imagine yourself in the future enjoying the advantages of consistent exercise, it encourages you to keep going even when things seem to be moving slowly.

By concentrating on the favorable outcomes you hope to attain, you create a mental picture that fortifies your determination. By giving your long-term objectives a more concrete and attainable sense, this hopeful vision may help you maintain your motivation.

Maintaining motivation and accountability is essential in any fitness program, particularly for senior citizens who want to improve their health by doing chair exercises. You can overcome obstacles, stay consistent, and accomplish your fitness goals while having fun if you have the right strategies in place.

Honoring Accomplishments

A good way to stay motivated on your fitness journey is to acknowledge and celebrate your victories, no matter how small. Setting goals helps you stay motivated and encourages the behaviors that lead to long-term success, whether you're using chair exercises to increase mobility, reduce weight, or regain your independence.

Beyond the health benefits, there are other reasons to celebrate your fitness achievements. Sustaining the emotional and mental drive necessary for sustained achievement is essential. *Here's why it's critical to acknowledge milestones:*

1. **Boosts Motivation:** When benefits, especially in fitness, take time to manifest, motivation may wane. Rewarding yourself for even small accomplishments, like completing a week of chair exercises or getting better posture, keeps you inspired to keep going.

2. **Boosts Confidence:** Many elderly people begin their fitness journey with doubts about their abilities, particularly if they haven't worked out in years or are recuperating from an illness. Celebrating every accomplishment demonstrates your capacity for growth and development. When you see

yourself succeeding at new things or reaching your objectives, your confidence increases.

3. **Reinforces Positive Behavior:** You can reward yourself for your efforts when you acknowledge your achievements. This creates a positive feedback loop that increases your likelihood of sticking to your habit by associating hard work with great feelings.

4. **Enhances Mental Health:** Exercise releases endorphins, which naturally elevate mood, but acknowledging and applauding achievements adds even more joy. Acknowledging your accomplishments enhances your mental health and lessens irritation, which can arise when you don't see results right away.

5. **Prevents Burnout:** When goals seem far or the road ahead seems lengthy, many people lose hope. You may prevent burnout by segmenting your exercise journey into smaller, more doable steps. You may prevent feeling overwhelmed by acknowledging and appreciating your progress at every stage.

Realistic Ideas For Honoring Success

The next step after recognizing your achievements is to rejoice. *Here are a few constructive and healthful methods to celebrate your achievements:*

1. **Establish mini-goals and treat yourself:** Divide your main exercise objectives into more manageable benchmarks. For instance, offer yourself a small reward at the end of each week, like a new book, a day off, or your favorite healthy treat, if your goal is to finish a 30-day chair exercise challenge.

2. **Create a Progress Journal:** Document your daily or weekly achievements in a journal. After working out, record your feelings, make any necessary adjustments, and consider your accomplishments. When you need motivation the most, going through your journal might give you a big lift.

3. **Celebrate with Others:** It can be satisfying to share your successes with loved ones, friends, or a fitness center. This helps you stay focused on your objectives and creates a supporting network around you. You might even inspire others to start their fitness journeys.

4. **Take Progress Pictures or Videos:** It can be motivating to see how far you've come. Take pictures or videos of yourself working out at different points during your journey. You will be reminded of your progress when you observe changes in your strength, flexibility, or posture.

5. **Treat Yourself to Fitness Equipment:** Think about rewarding yourself with new exercise gear as you reach significant life milestones. Your training routine might feel fresh and engaging with the addition of new shoes, resistance bands, or comfortable training apparel.

6. **Arrange a Special Outing:** Celebrate your successes by taking part in an enjoyable, wholesome activity. A peaceful spa day, a family outing to the park, or a nature stroll might all fall under this category. One of the best ways to reinforce the pleasant emotions associated with your hard work is to do something that brings you joy.

7. **Consider the Bigger Picture:** Sometimes just pausing to think about the broader picture is the greatest way to celebrate. Give yourself credit for taking charge of your health and acknowledge your improvement on all levels—physical, mental, and emotional. Keep in mind that the pursuit of health is a lifelong endeavor, and every accomplishment is a cause for celebration.

In addition to making your fitness journey more enjoyable, celebrating your accomplishments helps to guarantee long-term success. You're more likely to maintain your goals when you reward yourself for your accomplishments and hard work. This creates a never-ending circle of motivation, development, and fulfillment.

No matter how big or small, celebrating your accomplishments provides you the drive to keep going in the face of challenges.

CONCLUSION

As this masterpiece draws to a close, it's important to take a moment to consider all that you've learned and achieved so far. Even while chair exercises seem simple, they can have a big impact on your overall health and well-being. You've made a significant step toward a better, more active, and independent lifestyle by committing to these routines.

The importance of constancy is among the most important lessons to be learned from this book. Whether you want to improve your posture, boost your flexibility and mobility, acquire physical strength, or lose weight, consistency is key. As you age, chair exercises can help you maintain and perhaps improve your physical capabilities. You now know how to make fitness a regular part of your life by including these workouts in your everyday routine.

Exercise is more than just building muscle, especially as we become older. It's also about maintaining your mobility, freedom, and overall quality of life. Learning the exercises in this book is the first stage; the next step is to continue practicing them. Long-term advantages of this include gradual improvements in your strength, flexibility, balance, and general fitness.

Because their metabolisms and levels of physical activity fluctuate as they age, many seniors struggle to maintain a healthy weight. This book's chair exercises are a useful and secure way to help you reach your weight loss objectives. In addition to burning calories, these exercises increase muscle tone, which over time may increase metabolism.

Improving your whole health, not simply your appearance, is the goal of weight loss. Being overweight can cause mobility problems, increase your risk of heart disease, and put extra strain on your joints. You've given yourself the means to combat these health issues and enhance your general well-being by implementing the chair exercise regimens recommended in the book. Keep in mind that every workout contributes to the development of a healthier body and that even small efforts count.

One of the most crucial aspects of life as we get older is independence. In our youth, we often take for granted the ability to travel freely, carry out everyday tasks with ease, and navigate the world on our terms. However, many elderly people worry about losing their independence as their mobility deteriorates.

The purpose of the activities in this book is to assist you in regaining and preserving your freedom. You have the best chance to keep living your life as you see fit if you work on improving your strength, balance, and flexibility. As your muscles develop stronger and more coordinated, simple tasks like getting out of a chair, reaching for objects, and going upstairs become easier. Despite being simple and low-impact, these chair exercises can greatly improve your functional fitness, enabling you to carry on with your favorite activities independently.

The adaptability of chair exercises is one of their biggest benefits. Chair workouts can be customized to your current level of fitness, regardless of how long you've been exercising or how new you are. They are therefore an excellent option for seniors with varying skill levels. I've made adjustments and modifications throughout the book to ensure that everyone can participate, despite any physical limitations.

Wheelchair users and others with limited mobility are the target audience for the activities in this book. They emphasize vital areas including cardiovascular health, flexibility, and upper body strength. Everyone may benefit from a consistent fitness routine thanks to these exercises, which are made to provide great workouts while seated.

Remember that it's acceptable to start slowly and progressively raise the intensity over time if you ever feel that a certain workout is too tough. Growth, not perfection, is the aim. Pay attention to your body, understand your limits, and adjust your training regimen accordingly. Chair workouts are great because they can advance with you as your strength and mobility increase.

There are challenges unique to each fitness quest. It's important to recognize that obstacles are a normal part of the process, whether it's finding time to work out, managing health issues, or maintaining motivation in the face of hardship. The secret is to keep going even when things get tough.

One of the most motivating things about chair exercises is how they foster a sense of community. Chair exercises have become popular among seniors worldwide as a way to engage with people who share their goals and enhance their health. On this journey, you're not alone. Remember that you are part of a supportive network of people who are working toward the same goals, whether you attend local classes, participate in online organizations, or just tell your friends and family about your accomplishments.

Think of this book as a fresh start when you finish it. You will benefit greatly from the habits and exercises you have learned for the rest of your life. It is a continuous process that leads to improved mobility, independence, and health.

You've developed strength, confidence, and habits with these chair exercises that will help you in the years to come. Whether your goal is to stay active as you age, improve your mobility, or maintain your current level of fitness, the knowledge in this book will empower you to take charge of your health.

As you go along, refer to this book whenever you need guidance, inspiration, or encouragement. Regardless of age or fitness level, chair exercises are a long-term, effective way to maintain health and fitness. Your commitment to your health shows how strong, resilient, and determined you are.

I appreciate you for completing this great work. It's time to put what you've learned into practice and carry on leading the more independent, healthier life you deserve.